A GOLDEN TICKET TO YOUR DREAM BODY

HOW TO LOSE WEIGHT AND GET A FLAT TUMMY IN 7 DAYS WITHOUT EXERCISE

FATOKUN TEMITAYO

TABLE OF CONTENTS

INTRODUCTION

Are you tired of endless diets, grueling workouts, and slow progress? Do you dream of shedding those extra pounds quickly, without stepping foot in a gym? If so, you're not alone. Imagine waking up seven days from now, stepping onto the scale, and seeing a number that brings a smile to your face. You walk over to the mirror, lift your shirt, and there it is a flat tummy. No crunches, no planks, no hours spent on the treadmill. Just simple, effective strategies that have transformed your body in a week. Sounds too good to be true?

In a world where quick fixes and magic pills are the norm, it's easy to feel skeptical. But what if I told you that the secret to your dream body doesn't lie in exhausting workouts or restrictive diets? What if the key to lasting change was simpler than you ever imagined?

This research took me 9 months where I experimented myself as the guinea pig, and having achieved the desired results, I thought it to be the right time to share it with the world. This research was not just about weight loss, but also about making myself feel healthy and increasing my immunity and metabolism.

This book is not just another weight loss guide. It's a paradigm shift, a new way of thinking about health, body image, and self-love. It's about understanding that the journey to weight loss is not about punishing your body with grueling workouts, but about nourishing it, caring for it, and making small sustainable changes that add up to big results.

Each chapter of this book is designed to guide you through this process, providing practical tips, valuable insights, and effective strategies. You'll learn about the role of nutrition, the importance of hydration, the impact of sleep, and the power of mindset. You'll understand why dieting often fails and how a holistic approach can lead to lasting success.

The desire for rapid weight loss is universal, especially when an important event or beach vacation is looming. Remember, maintaining a healthy weight is not merely about fitting into a certain clothing size, it is about prioritizing one's health and well-being. From reducing the risk of chronic diseases to enhancing mental well-being and longevity, the benefits of weight management extend far beyond physical appearance.

So, are you ready to shed those stubborn pounds, boost your confidence, and feel lighter within a week?

Are you ready to challenge old beliefs, embrace new habits, and transform your body in just seven days? If the answer is yes, then let's get started.

CHAPTER 1

MINDSET AND INSPIRATION

What is Mindset?

Mindset alludes to perspectives, convictions, and suppositions that shape how we see the world and ourselves. Your mindset impacts your contemplations, feelings, and conducts and can essentially affect your outcome throughout everyday life, including weight reduction. This could be impacted by your way of life, the upsides of your family growing up, and the impact of your companions and friends.

There are two principal kinds of mindset:

Fixed Mindset

Development Mindset

A fixed mindset expects that our characteristics and capacities are foreordained and can't be changed. Individuals with a fixed mindset will generally surrender effectively when confronted with difficulties and accept that disappointment is an indication of inadequacy.

A development mindset accepts that our characteristics and capacities can be created through difficult work, practice, and diligence. Individuals with a development mindset embrace moves as any open doors to learn and improve and see disappointment as brief difficulties that can be survived.

What Mindset Means For Weight Reduction

Our mindset performs a basic part in our weight reduction venture. Here are a few ways by which mindset can influence weight reduction:

1. Inspiration

Inspiration is quite possibly the most basic variable that drives weight reduction achievement. Without inspiration, it tends to be trying to adhere to a good dieting plan, work-out consistently, and make other way of life changes fundamental for weight reduction. Your mindset can influence your inspiration levels. For instance, individuals with a development mindset are more persuaded to succeed in light of the fact that they view challenges as open doors to learn and get to the next level. They are not deterred by difficulties and disappointments; they use them as a growth opportunity to foster better techniques.

2. Self-Adequacy

Self-adequacy is the faith in your capacity to accomplish a particular objective. It is a basic consideration of weight reduction since, in such a case that you don't completely accept that you can get more fit, you are less inclined to invest the energy expected to accomplish your objectives. Individuals with a development mindset will generally have more elevated levels of self-adequacy since they accept their capacities can be created through exertion and perseverance. They are bound to adhere to their weight reduction plan in any event, when confronted with difficulties since they have faith in their capacity to conquer them.

3. Strength

Weight reduction is definitely not a direct cycle, and misfortunes are inescapable. Versatile individuals are better prepared to return from difficulties and proceed with their weight reduction venture. Versatility is firmly connected to mindset, with individuals with a development mindset being stronger than those with a fixed mindset. They can more readily adapt to misfortunes and disappointments since they view them as any open doors to learn and develop.

4. Self-Sympathy

Self-sympathy is treating oneself with generosity, understanding, and backing when confronted with troubles or mishaps. It is fundamental for practical weight reduction since it assists you with remaining persuaded and focused on your objectives in any event, when circumstances become difficult. Individuals with a development mindset will generally have more elevated levels of self-sympathy since they view mishaps and disappointments as a component of the educational experience. They are more lenient of themselves when they commit errors and are bound to utilize misfortunes to reconsider their methodology and move along.

Ways to Develop a Development Mindset for Weight Reduction

Now that we comprehend the work of mindset in practical weight reduction, we should investigate a ways to foster a development mindset to assist you with accomplishing your weight reduction objectives:

1. Embrace Difficulties

Rather than staying away from difficulties, embrace them as any open doors for development and learning.

Difficulties can assist you with creating flexibility, self-viability, and inspiration. When confronted with a test, ask yourself what you can gain from it and how you can utilize it to further develop your weight reduction system.

2. Center around Progress, not Perfection.

Many individuals get deterred when they don't see prompt outcomes from their weight reduction endeavors. Rather than zeroing in on flawlessness, center on progress. Commend each little triumph, whether a pound lost or a good dinner decision. Perceive that reasonable weight reduction requires some investment and exertion, and each little positive development is a bit nearer to your objective.

3. Practice Self-Sympathy

Be caring to yourself and practice self-sympathy. Keep away from self-fault and analysis when you commit an error or goof on your weight reduction plan. All things being equal, indulge you with thoughtfulness and understanding. Recall that difficulties are a characteristic piece of the weight reduction journey, and you can constantly begin again tomorrow.

4. Set Reasonable Objectives

Setting unreasonable objectives can prompt disappointment and demoralization. All things considered, lay out practical objectives that are feasible and quantifiable. Separate your objectives into more modest, more sensible advances and praise every achievement. This will assist you with remaining spurred and focused on your weight reduction plan.

5. Encircle Yourself with Energy.

Encircle yourself with individuals who support and energize your weight reduction venture. Keep away from pessimistic impacts and individuals who might attempt to sabotage your endeavors. Join a weight reduction support gathering or find a companion who shares your weight reduction objectives. Having an emotionally supportive network can assist you with remaining spurred and responsible.

Making a Triumphant Mindset for Weight Reduction

Practical weight reduction is a journey that requires a solid mindset. Your mindset can influence your inspiration, self-adequacy, strength, and self-sympathy, basic for weight reduction achievement. Developing a development mindset can assist you with conquering difficulties, remain roused, and accomplish weight reduction objectives. Embrace difficulties center around progress, practice self-empathy, set sensible objectives, and encircle yourself with energy. Keep in mind, practical weight reduction is a long distance race, not a run, and each positive development is a bit nearer to your objective.

CHAPTER 2

NUTRITION STRATEGIES

Making a Nutrition Plan

Eating great plays a significant part in weight reduction and maintenance. A triumphant methodology for weight reduction incorporates both caloric limitation and sufficient activity while calories are essential for weight control, it's excessively tight to imagine that energy-in and energy-out is the main element to think about in weight reduction. These variables are likewise involved:

- Climate
- Ailments
- Active work levels
- Prescriptions
- Financial aspects
- Hereditary qualities

- Hormone

- Psychological wellness

- Sleep

Your smartest way is to work with a medical care proficient for a customized weight reduction plan. In the event that is preposterous, you can follow the overall data in the Dietary Rules for Americans about the work of nourishment in weight reduction. It suggests a differed diet that incorporates:

- Vegetables and organic product

- Grains (counting entire grains)

- Protein food varieties

- Dairy

- Oils

The sum (segment) of food that you ought to eat is well defined for your ongoing weight and your weight reduction objectives. Regardless of whether you cut back on calories, it is essential to eat various food sources to get the entirety of the protein, solid fats, nutrients, and minerals that your body requires. Zeroing in on viewpoints past food is additionally essential. Actual work, hydration, sleep, and different parts are completely interconnected in your weight reduction venture.

Meal Planning

Your body requires supplements consistently so it works appropriately. The Dietary Rules were intended to guarantee that supplement needs are met with various food varieties including vegetables, natural products, protein, and grains.

You can design meals utilizing the five food techniques. At the point when you plan meals, consider these plate extents:

1. Make around 50% of your plate vegetables and natural products.

2. Make a quarter of your plate grains. Pick entire grains to some degree half of the time.

3. Make a quarter of your plate protein from food varieties like poultry, fish, eggs, meat, vegetables, nuts, and seeds.7

4. Have a serving of calcium-rich food varieties like milk, soy refreshment, or yogurt.

The specific measure of food you will require relies upon your objectives. As well as eating all the more entire food sources like vegetables, you can likewise scale back vigorously handled food varieties like inexpensive food, bundled snacks, prepared merchandise, and candy.

A straightforward meal plan might seem to be this. You can repeat this 5-day plan multiple times to finish a 30-day plan.

Day 1

Breakfast: Plain Greek yogurt with strawberries and low-sugar (3 grams of sugar or less per serving), oat-based granola

Nibble: Almonds and grapes

Lunch: Fish soften sandwich with cheddar and tomatoes on entire grain bread, presented with carrots, red peppers, and an apple as an afterthought

Nibble: Cucumber and hummus

Supper: Chicken with earthy colored rice and pan-seared vegetables.

Day 2

Breakfast: Chia pudding with Greek yogurt and organic product

Nibble: cheddar and an apple

Lunch: Jab bowl: fish (or tofu) with earthy colored rice, blended vegetables, kelp and sesame seeds

Nibble: Trail blend

Supper: Pesto shrimp and broccoli served over entire grain pasta

Day 3

Breakfast: Pounded avocado and ricotta cheddar on entire grain toast with a side of berries

Nibble: New peach, granola, and Greek yogurt

Lunch: Turkey sandwich with lettuce, tomato and sweet peppers; banana

Nibble: Plain popcorn

Supper: Chickpea and cauliflower curry with quinoa

Day 4

Breakfast: Cereal with banana, peanut butter, and soy or cow's milk

Nibble: Hummus and carrots

Lunch: Dark bean and cheddar burrito in entire grain tortilla, with lettuce, tomato, sweet peppers, and avocado

Nibble: Plain popcorn

Supper: Sautéed chicken and blended vegetables on soba noodles

Day 5

Breakfast: Fried eggs, entire grain toast, and tomato

Nibble: Medjool dates with peanut butter or almond spread

Lunch: Chicken Caesar salad with parmesan cheddar and bread garnishes in addition to a pear

Nibble: Little part of your #1 frozen yogurt

Supper: Lemon-margarine halibut with green beans and potatoes

CHAPTER 3

HYDRATION AND DETOXIFICATION

The Connection between Hydration and Weight Reduction

Does drinking water assist you with getting in shape?

With regards to weight reduction, the significance of hydration can't be adequately featured. Water plays a critical part in our digestion, supporting the breakdown and dispersion of supplements in our body. It likewise assists with stifling hunger, causing us to feel fuller and diminishing the probability of gorging. Nonetheless, it's essential to take note that while water can aid weight reduction; it's anything but an enchanted arrangement. A decent eating routine and normal activity is as yet key parts of any fruitful weight reduction plan.

On the other side, lack of hydration can obstruct your weight reduction endeavors. At the point when the body is dried out, it can't work at its ideal. This incorporates dialing back the digestion, which can prompt weight gain or trouble getting in shape. Also, drying out can frequently is confused with hunger, prompting superfluous calorie utilization. In any case, likewise the importance of drinking unreasonable measures of water isn't valuable and can prompt water inebriation, a difficult condition. In this way, it's essential to find some kind of harmony and guarantee you're drinking a proper measure of water for your body and action level.

How Does Drinking Water Cause You To Get More fit?

Remaining very much hydrated is a pivotal part of a sound digestion. Drinking water helps increment your body's capacity to consume calories, an interaction known as thermo genesis. During thermo genesis, your body utilizes energy to warm the water to internal heat level, consequently consuming calories. This metabolic lift can be especially gainful for weight reduction.

Reliable hydration likewise helps with absorption. Water is fundamental for the legitimate working of the gastrointestinal lot. It helps separate food with the goal that your body can retain the supplements. This cycle can assist with forestalling clogging and keep your stomach related framework chugging along as expected, adding to a better digestion.

How much water to drink to get in shape?

Expect to drink no less than eight 8-ounce glasses of water a day. Not exclusively will this assist with keeping your digestion working ideally, yet it can likewise assist with controlling your hunger. Frequently, sensations of yearning are indications of drying out. Thus, prior to going after snacks, take a stab at drinking a glass of water first. You could find that it controls your desires and assists you with remaining focused with your weight reduction objectives.

The Effect of Water on Craving and Calorie Consumption

Drinking water can essentially influence your craving and calorie consumption. Research has demonstrated the way that polishing off water before a meal can prompt a decrease in how much calories are drunk during the meal. This is fundamentally on the grounds that water occupies room in the stomach, prompting a sensation of completion and lessening hunger. A review directed on grown-ups found that the people who hydrated before their meal lost 44% more weight than the individuals who didn't.

Also, replacing fatty drinks like pop and squeeze with water can additionally help in lessening your general calorie consumption. Water has zero calories and can give the sensation of completion without adding additional calories. This makes it a fantastic instrument for weight the board. It's additionally significant that the body frequently mistakes hunger for hunger. Thus, remaining hydrated enough can forestall gorging brought about by this distortion of the body's requirements.

Water's Part in Detoxification and Weight Reduction

Quite possibly the main way that water adds to weight reduction is through its part in detoxification. Water supports flushing out toxins from the body, which works on general wellbeing as well as improves digestion. A proficient digestion is essential for consuming fat and calories, along these lines working with weight reduction. Besides, poisons can frequently prompt bulging and water maintenance, which can add to your weight. By assisting with disposing of these poisons, water can in this way assist in diminishing with weighting.

One more perspective to consider is the work of water in processing. Legitimate hydration is fundamental for ideal assimilation and supplement retention. At the point when the body has dried out, it can't actually separate food or assimilate supplements. This can prompt a more slow digestion and weight gain. Then again, remaining all around hydrated can keep your stomach related framework chugging along as expected, which can help with weight reduction.

How much water would it be advisable for you to drink to shed pounds?

- Drink no less than 8 glasses of water a day
- Drink a glass of water before every meal
- Supplant sweet beverages with water
- Hydrate at whatever point you feel hungry

The Advantages of Drinking Water Before Meals for Weight Reduction

Incorporating a basic propensity for drinking water before a meal can essentially add to your weight reduction venture. This training supports upgrading satiety, which thus, can assist you with consuming fewer calories during your meal. Research shows that drinking around 17 ounces of water can build your metabolic rate by 30% in sound people.

This metabolic lift happens in the span of 10 minutes of water utilization and arrives at a maximum after around 30-40 minutes. Moreover, drinking water before meals makes a feeling of completion, prompting a decrease in how much food is polished off. This is a helpful technique for those meaning to shed pounds, as it is a characteristic and solid method for confining caloric consumption.

Step by Step Instructions to Integrate More Water into Your Everyday Eating Regimen

Expanding your everyday water consumption can be accomplished through different strategies. Conveying a water bottle with you over the course of the day is a reasonable and helpful method for guaranteeing you're drinking enough. This not just fills in as a steady suggestion to hydrate yet in addition permits you to follow your utilization. In any case, it's critical to take note of that while expanding water consumption can support weight reduction; it shouldn't supplant a reasonable eating routine and normal activity.

Another compelling strategy is to drink fruit sources with high water content. Fruits grown from the ground like cucumbers, watermelon, and oranges can altogether add to your hydration levels. This approach has the additional advantage of giving fundamental nutrients and supplements. On the drawback, depending entirely on high-water food sources for hydration can prompt a more fatty consumption, so keeping a reasonable diet is significant.

CHAPTER 4

SLEEP AND STRESS MANAGEMENT

The Connection between Sleep, Stress, and Weight Reduction

Research has shown that there are areas of strength between sleep, stress, and weight reduction. The absence of sleep can prompt an expansion in hunger hormones, making it harder to control desires and eat a solid eating routine. Stress can likewise prompt weight gain by setting off the arrival of the hormone cortisol, which can cause an expansion in craving. By tending to sleep and stress management, we can further develop weight reduction endeavors and generally speaking wellbeing and prosperity.

The Significance of Sleep in Weight Reduction

Sleep assumes a significant part in weight reduction by managing hormones that control yearning and digestion. Satisfactory sleep is important for the legitimate working of the hormone leptin and ghrelin, which control sensations of craving and healthy diet. At the point when we don't get sufficient sleep, levels of ghrelin (the hormone that invigorates hunger) increase, while levels of leptin (the hormone that stifles craving) decrease, making it harder to control desires and eats a sound eating routine. Also, absence of rest can prompt diminished digestion, which can cause it to be more challenging to consume calories and get thinner.

Conversation of the Impact of Lack of Sleep on Weight Gain

Ongoing lack of sleep can prompt weight gain in more ways than one. One of the primary ways is by affecting the hormone that controls hunger, as examined previously. Restless individuals will generally pine for fatty food sources and devour more calories by and large, which can prompt weight gain.

Ways to Further Develop Sleep Habits

To further develop sleep habits, it is essential to lay out an ordinary sleep plan, keep away from caffeine and hardware near sleep time, and make a loosening up sleep time schedule. Moreover, making a cool, dim, and calm climate can assist with working on the nature of sleep. Practice unwinding strategies like yoga, reflection, or profound breathing can assist with lessening feelings of anxiety before bed. It's additionally essential to keep away from huge meals and animating exercises near sleep time and to ensure your bed and pillow are agreeable.

The Significance of Stress Management in Weight Reduction

Stress can assume a significant part in weight reduction by setting off the arrival of the hormone cortisol, which can cause an expansion in hunger. At the point when we're under pressure, cortisol levels rise and can cause desires for unhealthy, sweet food varieties. Furthermore, stress can prompt profound eating and can make it harder to adhere to a solid eating regimen and exercise plan.

Conversation of the Impact of Constant Stress on Weight Gain

Ongoing pressure can prompt weight gain in more than one way. As referenced above, cortisol, the pressure hormone can cause an expansion in hunger and desires for fatty food varieties. Furthermore, when we're under pressure, we will generally take part in ways of behaving like gorging, skipping meals, and ignoring actual work. Over the long haul, these ways of behaving can prompt weight gain. Stress can likewise upset sleep, which can additionally add to weight gain.

Methodologies for Overseeing Pressure and Advancing Unwinding

There are a few methodologies for overseeing pressure that can assist with weight reduction. A few compelling strategies incorporate profound breathing, contemplation, yoga, and exercise. Furthermore, journaling, conversing with a specialist, or investing energy with friends and family can likewise be useful. Finding a pressure easing movement that you appreciate and creating it a customary piece of your routine can be compelling in overseeing feelings of anxiety.

Joining Sleep and Stress Management for Weight Reduction

Sleep and stress management are firmly interconnected and are both vital for weight reduction. Sufficient sleep is vital for the legitimate working of hormones that control appetite and digestion while stress management can assist with forestalling gorging and close-to-home eating. By tending to both sleep and stress, you will actually want to all the more likely control your cravings, increase your energy levels, and further develop your general prosperity.

Tips for Making a Decent and Economical Weight Reduction Plan that Incorporate Sleep and Stress Management

To make a weight reduction plan that incorporates sleep and stress management, it's vital to lay out normal sleep and wake times, lay out a sleep time schedule, and ensure your rest climate is agreeable. Moreover, it's essential to find pressure easing exercises that you appreciate, set aside a few minutes for them consistently, and attempt to stay away from or limit exercises that cause pressure.

CHAPTER 5

DIGESTION BOOSTER

How Does Digestion Function?

Basically, your digestion is a substance process that converts starches, proteins, and fats from your food into the energy that your cells need to work.

Your metabolic rate is how much time it takes your body to process and consume energy, or calories, from the food you eat. Your basal metabolic rate (BMR) is how much energy or calories your body needs to keep up with fundamental capabilities while you're resting. It's the number of calories that you would have to make if you never moved.

Your BMR represents around 70% of your day to day energy use.

A Few Things That Impact Your BMR:

- **Hereditary qualities:** The Calories you consume each day are still up in the air by hereditary qualities.

- **Age:** Your typical BMR diminishes by 2% each ten years after age 20.

- **Orientation:** Men will generally have a higher BMR than ladies.

- **Weight:** As your weight increments, so does your BMR.

- **Level:** Tall individuals will generally have a higher BMR than more diminutive individuals.

- **Body Makeup:** Your BMR will be higher assuming you have more muscle and less fat.

- **Diet:** Long haul low-calorie admission can fundamentally diminish your BMR. Thus, outrageous slimming down can neutralize you.

Certain clinical issues, certain meds, and environment can likewise change your BMR.

The amount you move, both overall and with work out, likewise mirrors the absolute number of calories you consume. You likewise consume calories processing food, an interaction called diet-prompted thermo genesis.

Do Digestion Boosters Work?

A few organizations sell items that evidently support your digestion. Most cases they do this through a cycle called thermo genesis, or expanded heat creation. This interaction invigorates energy use and can expand your digestion and assist with consuming calories.

Most enhancements that cause your digestion contain a blend of fixings. Since these fixings are quite often tried independently, we really want to evaluate them on that premise.

How about we investigate the absolute most normal fixings tracked down in supplements that help to increase digestion?

Caffeine

Research has demonstrated the way that caffeine can increment thermo genesis.

Six unique researchers have found that individuals consume more calories when they take a base everyday portion of 270 milligrams (mg) of caffeine.

To place that in context, most caffeine supplements contain 200 mg of caffeine, while one mug of espresso contains around 95 mg. notwithstanding, assuming you drink caffeine routinely, this impact may be reduced.

Converse with your PCP prior to adding more caffeine to your eating routine. Also, ensure your caffeine sources aren't excessively high in calories. In the event that you drink too many improved espresso drinks or chai tea, you could end up putting on weight!

Capsaicin

Capsaicin is the compound that puts the hot in jalapeños. There's some sign it might assist with advancing weight reduction.

Capsaicin can expand how much calories you consume by roughly 50 calories every day. Those calories can accumulate after some time, adding to long haul weight reduction. So consider flavoring it up in your kitchen!

L-carnitine

L-carnitine is a substance that assists your body with transforming fat into energy. While your body produces it in your liver and kidneys, you can likewise track it in meat, dairy items, nuts, and vegetables.

L-carnitine may assist with treating a few circumstances, including coronary illness, fringe conduit infection, and diabetic neuropathy.

Chromium picolinate

Chromium is a mineral that your body involves in modest quantities. Chromium picolinate supplements are valuable for individuals who have a lack of chromium.

Formed linoleic corrosive (CLA)

Likewise with many enhancements, research shows that CLA might advance weight reduction and fat misfortune, yet the impacts are little and questionable.

Gastrointestinal issues and weakness are normal symptoms of taking CLA supplements, so you might need to pass on this one.

Green tea

Various researches has been led on the adequacy of green tea for weight reduction. Few have revealed critical outcomes.

One review uncovers that catechins and caffeine found in green tea might assist with supporting weight upkeep.

Green tea is viewed as a protected expansion to the vast majority's eating regimens.

Resveratrol

Resveratrol is a substance found in the skin of red grapes, mulberries, Japanese knotweed, and peanuts. Studies recommend it consumes fat in rodents.

You can check more supplements for weight loss here to purchase directly. Keep in mind; look for proficient clinical counsel prior to consuming the medications so you can get an enhancement that is reasonable for your well-being.

CHAPTER 6

MEAL PLAN FOR 7 DAYS

7-Day Sample Weight Reduction and Flat Tummy Plan

This one-week meal plan was intended for around 2,000 individual calories each day yet meant to accomplish weight reduction and flat tummy through consumption of 1,500 to 1,750 calories each day with 3 meals and 2 snacks. Your everyday calorie objective might shift. Realize what it is beneath, and then make changes to the arrangement to accommodate your particular requirements. Consider working with an enrolled dietitian or talking with one more medical care supplier to precisely evaluate and make arrangements for your dietary necessities more.

To advance weight reduction, this plan is low-carb, high protein, and moderate-fat. The macronutrient proportions of this meal plan are 25% sugars, 40% protein, and 35% dietary fat. Food swap or replacement is fine the same way as you do with comparative menu things and piece sizes.

Day 1

Breakfast

- 3 huge fried eggs
- 1 cut entire wheat toast

Micronutrients: 350 calories, 21 grams protein, 17 grams starches, and 21 grams fat

Nibble

- 1 little compartment (5.3 ounces) of plain nonfat Greek Yogurt
- 1/4 cup blueberries
- 1-ounce cashew pieces

Micronutrients: 272 calories, 20 grams protein, 20 grams starches, and 14 grams fat

Lunch

- 4 ounces barbecued chicken bosom
- 2 cups cleaved romaine lettuce
- 1/4 cup cut strawberries
- 2 tablespoons sunflower seeds
- 1 tablespoon olive oil
- 1 tablespoon balsamic vinegar

Micronutrients: 418 calories, 38 grams of protein, 11 grams of starches, and 26 grams of fat

Nibble

- 1 scoop whey protein powder blended in 1 cup nonfat milk

Micronutrients: 193 calories, 28 grams of protein, 18 grams of carbs, and 1 gram of fat

Supper

- 4 ounces barbecued sirloin steak
- 1 little prepared potato
- 1 cup steamed blended vegetables

Micronutrients: 449 calories, 36 grams of protein, 39 grams of starches, and 17 grams of fat

Day to day Aggregates: 1,683 calories, 144 grams protein, 106 grams carbs, and 79 grams fat.

Day 2

Breakfast

- 1/3 cup dry oats (cook in water and a sprinkle of salt and cinnamon)
- 4 huge fried egg whites
- 1 ounce fragmented almonds

Micronutrients: 340 calories, 24 grams protein, 25 grams carbs, and 17 grams fat

Nibble

- 1 medium apple

- 2 tablespoons regular peanut butter

Micronutrients: 316 calories, 9 grams of protein, 38 grams of starches, and 17 grams of fat

Lunch

- 4 ounces strong white fish in water (depleted)
- 1 tablespoon olive oil mayonnaise
- 16 slight wheat saltines

Micronutrients: 327 calories, 29 grams of protein, 22 grams of starches, and 13 grams of fat

Nibble

- 1 scoop whey protein powder blended in espresso or water
- 1-ounce almonds

Micronutrients: 280 calories, 26 grams protein, 12 grams carbs, and 16 grams fat

Supper

- 6 ounces barbecued chicken bosom
- 1 cup steamed broccoli

Micronutrients: 306 calories, 54 grams protein, 11 grams carbs, and 6 grams fat

Day to day Aggregates: 1,569 calories, 141 grams protein, 108 grams carbs, and 70 grams fat

Day 3

Breakfast

- 6 ounces 2% curds
- 1/4 cup pineapple pieces
- 1-ounce cashew pieces

Micronutrients: 337 calories, 22 grams of protein, 27 grams of carbs, and 17 grams of fat

Nibble

- 1/2 cup guacamole

- 1 red chime pepper, cut

Micronutrients: 213 calories, 3 grams protein, 18 grams carbs, and 17 grams fat

Lunch

- 6 ounces of broiled turkey store meat
- 1 cut of provolone cheddar
- 1 (6-7 inch) flour tortilla or wrap

Micronutrients: 340 calories, 43 grams protein, 15 grams carbs, and 12 grams fat

Nibble

- 1 cup salted and arranged edamame in the unit
- 1 cup cut carrots

Micronutrients: 238 calories, 20 grams protein, 25 grams starches, and 8 grams fat

Supper

- 6-ounce 97% lean ground meat burger

- 1 slider-size burger bun
- 2 cuts tomato
- 2 lettuce leaves
- 1 tablespoon ketchup
- 2 cuts red onion

Micronutrients: 432 calories, 54 grams protein, 25 grams carbs, and 11 grams fat

Day to day Aggregates: 1,559 calories, 143 grams protein, 110 grams starches, and 65 grams fat

Day 4

Breakfast

- 1 serving Oats Curds Waffles
- 1/2 cup raspberries

Micronutrients: 262 calories, 21 grams protein, 21 grams carbs, and 11 grams fat

Nibble

- 2 huge hard-bubbled eggs

- 1 section skim mozzarella string cheddar

- 1 cup grapes

- 1 cup cut carrots

Micronutrients: 359 calories, 21 grams of protein, 41 grams of starches, and 14 grams of fat

Lunch

- 6 ounces barbecued chicken bosom

- 2 cups romaine lettuce

- 1/4 cup corn bits

- 1/4 cup dark beans

- 1/4 avocado

- 1 tablespoon lime juice

- 1 tablespoon olive oil

- 1 tablespoon cleaved cilantro

Micronutrients: 562 calories, 57 grams protein, 26 grams starches, and 28 grams fat

Nibble

- 1 scoop whey protein powder blended in espresso or water

Micronutrients: 110 calories, 20 grams of protein, 6 grams of starches, and 1 gram of fat

Supper

- 6 ounces almost 100% sans fat ground turkey bosom, sauteed in 1 teaspoon olive oil and blended in with 1/4 cup marinara sauce
- 2 cups steamed zucchini noodles

Micronutrients: 284 calories, 40 grams protein, 12 grams starches, and 9 grams fat

Day to day Aggregates: 1,578 calories, 159 grams protein, 107 grams carbs, and 63 grams fat

Day 5

Breakfast

Smoothie: 1 scoop whey protein powder, 1 little frozen banana, 1 tablespoon peanut butter, 1 cup nonfat milk, ice

Micronutrients: 383 calories, 34 grams protein, 45 grams carbs, and 10 grams fat

Nibble

- 1/4 cup pistachios, in the shell

Micronutrients: 175 calories, 6.5 grams protein, 8 grams starches, and 14 grams fat

Lunch

- 4 ounces store cook meat
- 1 cut of provolone cheddar
- 1 cut of rye bread
- 2 cuts red onion
- 2 cuts tomato

Micronutrients: 337 calories, 34 grams of protein, 18 grams of starches, and 11 grams of fat

Nibble

- 1 little holder (5.3 ounces) of plain nonfat Greek Yogurt
- 1-ounce almonds

Micronutrients: 258 calories, 21 grams of protein, 11 grams of starches, and 15 grams of fat

Supper

- 4 ounces barbecued chicken bosom
- 1/2 cup cooked earthy colored rice
- 1 tablespoon margarine
- 1 cup steamed blended vegetables

Micronutrients: 424 calories, 38 grams of protein, 33 grams of starches, and 17 grams of fat

Day to day Aggregates: 1,578 calories, 133 grams protein, 115 grams carbs, and 68 grams fat

Day 6

Breakfast

Short-term Oats: Consolidate the accompanying in a bowl, cover, and refrigerate for the time being. Top with 1 ounce of hacked pecans.

- 1/3 cup dry oats
- 2 ounces plain nonfat Greek yogurt
- 1 scoop whey protein powder
- run salt
- 1/4 cup nonfat milk
- Run of cinnamon

Micronutrients: 464 calories, 34 grams of protein, 38 grams of starches, and 22 grams of fat

Nibble

- 1 cup salted and arranged edamame, in the case
- 1 cup cut carrots

Micronutrients: 238 calories, 20 grams protein, 25 grams carbs, and 8 grams fat

Lunch

Quesadilla: 3 ounces barbecued chicken bosom, 1/4 cup destroyed Mexican cheddar, and 1 (6-7 inch) flour tortilla; present with 2 tablespoons salsa

Micronutrients: 306 calories, 37 grams of protein, 17 grams of carbs, and 11 grams of fat

Nibble

- 6 ounces 2% curds
- 1 medium peach

Micronutrients: 196 calories, 19 grams protein, 22 grams carbs, and 4 grams fat

Supper

- 6 ounces barbecued salmon
- 6 huge steamed asparagus lances

Micronutrients: 370 calories, 40 grams protein, 3 grams starches, and 21 grams fat

Day to day Aggregates: 1,573 calories, 149 grams protein, 107 grams starches, and 67 grams fat

Day 7

Breakfast

- 4 egg white omelet with 1/4 cup cut mushrooms, 1 cup spinach, and 1/4 avocado
- 1 cut of wheat toast

Micronutrients: 250 calories, 20 grams protein, 23 grams starches, and 8 grams fat

Nibble

Smoothie: 2/3 cup plain nonfat Greek Yogurt, 1 cup nonfat milk, 1/4 cup frozen blueberries, 1/4 cup frozen strawberries, 3 tablespoons hemp seeds, 1/2 frozen banana

Micronutrients: 425 calories, 34 grams of protein, 42 grams of starches, and 16 grams of fat

Lunch

- 6 ounces barbecued salmon
- 6 steamed asparagus lances

Micronutrients: 370 calories, 40 grams protein, 3 grams carbs, and 21 grams fat

Nibble

2 hard-bubbled eggs

Micronutrients: 155 calories, 13 grams of protein, 1 gram of carbs, and 11 grams of fat

Supper

- 4 ounces barbecued chicken bosom
- 1 cup steamed pan sear vegetables
- 1/2 cup cooked white rice
- 1 tablespoon teriyaki sauce

Micronutrients: 457 calories, 43 grams of protein, 40 grams of carbs, and 15 grams of fat

Day to day Aggregates: 1,657 calories, 150 grams protein, 110 grams starches, and 71 grams fat

Tips On the Best Way to Meal Plan for a Weight Reduction Diet

1. Decide your calorie needs. Begin by sorting out the number of calories that you need to eat each day by utilizing an everyday calorie mini-computer. From that point, decide the number of grams of protein, carbs, and fats by utilizing macronutrient proportions like the ones shared previously. Partition those numbers by how much meals and snacks to decide segment sizes.

2. Record what you need to eat. Take a couple of seconds to make a rundown of meals and snacks you'd like to eat. Plug those into the week ahead to make a meal plan.

3. Use extras. Make an additional piece at supper so you can have it for lunch the following day. That way you're investing less energy in cooking.

4. Make it a point to reorder days. It's alright to eat exactly the same thing once in a while, as a matter of

fact; doing so can make your life more straightforward. You realize you like the food and there's less thought expected to sort out the thing you will eat.

5. Stock your fridge and storeroom. Shop ahead of time for the food varieties you want on your meal plan that the way you're constantly arranged when supper time comes.

6. Prepare meals before the night whenever the situation allows. Making food the prior night can save opportunity in the first part of the day while you're hurrying to get out the entryway. What's more, when you get back home from a seemingly endless workday, the last thing you maintain that you should do is cook. A prepared meal makes it simple to warm up when it is time to eat.

CHAPTER 7

LIFESTYLE HACKS

1. Know where you are beginning. Keep a food record for three days. Track all the food and drinks you eat alongside the parts. Recognize how frequently you are eating away from home, eating takeout or purchasing food on the run.

2. Set your objective and make a plan. What is your objective? Would you like to shed pounds to work on your wellbeing? Do you fantasize about squeezing into an old set of pants? How might you accomplish your objective? Will you cook more meals at home? Will you eat more modest bits? Be explicit and begin little.

3. Distinguish hindrances to your objectives and ways of conquering them. Might a bustling timetable at some

point impede going to the exercise center? Get up an hour sooner. Has a vacant storage space kept you from cooking at home? Look into a few solid recipes, then, at that point, go to the supermarket for a rundown of ingredients you'll have to set them up.

4. Distinguish current propensities that lead to unhealthful eating. Do you unwind and remunerate yourself by eating before the television? Do you skip lunch just to feel starved by midafternoon, prepared to eat anything in sight? Do you complete all that on your plate even after you begin to feel full?

5. Control your bits. Refamiliarize yourself with standard serving sizes. Did you have any idea that one serving of poultry or meat is 4 ounces, or the size of a deck of playing a game of cards? Or on the other hand that one serving of pasta is just 1/2 cup?

6. Recognize appetite and satiety signals. Know about physical versus profound yearning. Do you eat when you feel something actual in your body that answers food? Or on the other hand do you eat when you are worried,

exhausted, drained, miserable, or restless? Attempt to quit eating Prior to getting full (it requires around 20 minutes for your mind to enroll "quit eating" signals from your stomach). Food sources that can assist you with feeling more full incorporate high-fiber food varieties like vegetables, entire grains, beans, and vegetables; protein (fish, poultry, eggs); and water.

7. Center on the positive changes. Changing conduct takes time, something like three months. Try not to surrender in the event that you goof en route. Get support from others and find opportunities to recognize the progressions you have made.

8. Go with the 80/20 rule. Keep focused 80% of the time; however leave some space for a couple of guilty pleasures. You would rather not feel denied or remorseful.

9. Center on in general wellbeing. Walk, dance, bicycle, rake leaves, garden, and find exercises you appreciate and do them consistently. Ditch the "diet" path and spotlight on occasional, entire, excellent food varieties.

10. Eat gradually and carefully. Partake in the whole experience of eating. Carve out an opportunity to see the value in the fragrances, tastes, and surfaces of the dinner before you.

11. Stay Hydrated

We've shrouded this in the past part, however, it merits underscoring. Appropriate hydration upholds absorption, digestion, and by and large wellbeing:

- Convey a Water Jug: Keep water reachable over the course of the day.
- Mix Your Water: Add lemon, cucumber, or mint for some extra zing.

12. Morning Herbal Routine: Taste chamomile, mint, or ginger tea with lemon. Picture each cup as an elixir. Chamomile calms pressure, mint animates ginger lights your internal heater, and lemon supports absorption and assists with lessening weight.

13. Outlook and Visualization

Your outlook impacts your activities. Utilize these methods:

- Confirmations: Rehash positive explanations like "I'm equipped for accomplishing my objectives."

- Picture Achievement: Envision yourself with a slim body and flat tummy, feel the certainty.

14. Stay away from Late-Evening food

Late-evening eating frequently prompts weight gain. Carry out these methodologies:

- Set a Deadline: Try not to eat following a specific hour (e.g., 8 PM).

- Clean Your Teeth: After supper, clean your teeth to flag that eating time is finished.

15. Consider periodic fasting.

Numerous researches on the benefits of intermittent fasting have shown that it can indeed aid in weight loss. It can help you burn fatter in a day by increasing your metabolism in addition to helping you limit your calorie intake. While there are many health advantages to fasting, such as lowered blood pressure and improved heart health, some people doubt the long-term viability of this weight loss strategy.

CHAPTER 8

TRACKING PROGRESS

Tracking Progress is an indispensable piece of this journey. It gives inspiration, keeps up with focus, and takes into consideration acclimations to the arrangement depending on the plan.

Why Track Progress?

Tracking Progress is fundamental because of multiple factors:

1. **Inspiration:** Seeing substantial outcomes can extraordinarily rouse. At the point when you keep tabs on your development, you can perceive how far you've come, which can urge you to continue onward.

2. Responsibility: Regular Tracking can consider you responsible for your objectives. It fills in as a sign of what you're making progress toward and why.

3. Distinguishing Examples: Tracking can assist with recognizing examples or patterns. For instance, you could see that you will quite often lose more weight when you hydrate or get more rest.

4. Adapting: On the off chance that you're not seeing the outcomes you need, Tracking Progress can assist you with sorting out what changes should be made. Perhaps you really want to change your eating regimen or make changes to your way of life.

Understanding Body Weight Rate

A gauging scale might fill you in regarding your total body mass, which might incorporate muscle mass, body fat, and weight of the relative multitude of essential organs in the body. Be that as it may, a muscle to fat ratio just uncovers how much fat you have in the body.

Estimating your muscle versus fat ratio assists you with following the all out fat in your body, yet doesn't ascertain the muscle mass.

In correlation, Body Mass Index (BMI) considers both your height and weight. Specialists use BMI estimations to check whether an individual is overweight, underweight stout, or of typical weight. In any case, this technique doesn't give the whole picture.

For example, an athlete or a bodybuilder might have more bulk than is common for his weight, which is the reason BMI estimation might proclaim him as overweight, regardless of whether he has low muscle to fat ratio. All things considered, computing muscle versus fat ratio is said to convey more precise outcomes in following endlessly weight reduction progress.

How to Calculate Body Fat Percentage

There are multiple ways of computing and measuring your body fat ratio. These include:

1. Muscle to fat ratio calipers (Skin fold calipers) - Skin fold calipers include estimating the thickness of the subcutaneous fat. Typically, the chest, abs, and thighs are the three spots utilized for the estimation cycle.

2. Submerged gauging - It is accepted that submerged, the fat ascents and floats while the lean tissue sinks, which gives one an exact gauge of the muscle to fat ratio synthesis.

3. The Body Case - a gadget utilizes air dislodging to quantify your weight, volume, and thickness and computes your muscle versus fat ratio. This technique is pricey.

4. Double X-beam absorptiometry (DEXA) check - This strategy is thought of as exceptionally exact since it takes a full double X-beam of your body creation and gives you numbers.

Estimations can help (Abdomen to-Hip Proportion)

The midsection to-hip proportion is an extraordinary method for monitoring your weight. It is likewise a technique utilized by clinical experts to see whether overabundance weight is seriously endangering an individual's wellbeing.

To follow midriff-to-hip proportion, you really want to gauge the proportion of your abdomen outline to your hip circuit. For example, partition your midriff periphery by your hip boundary.

As per the World Wellbeing Association (WHO), a moderate WHR in men is 0.9 or less and for ladies, it is 0.85 or less. A WHR of 1.0 or higher makes all kinds of people inclined to coronary illness and different circumstances related to being overweight.

Observe how your clothes fit you

One more simple and cost-accommodating method for deciding your weight reduction progress is by observing the way that your clothes fit you. Snap a photo of yourself toward the beginning of your weight reduction journey and continue to accept new pictures as and when you believe you have hit another achievement. This way you will realize the amount of progress you have made.

Moreover, you can try on your clothes to continue to keep tabs on your development. Toward the start of the journey, wear something somewhat close to your body and continue to attempt it at regular intervals to take note of the distinction. Contingent upon how they fit, you can decide if you have gained ground.

Take Progress Photographs

Visual proof is strong. Take pictures toward the start of your journey and intermittently from there on:

- Front View: Stand straight, arms loose.

- Side View: Profile photograph to follow changes in your waistline.

- Back View: Catch your advancement from all the angles.

Taking photographs of yourself from various points can give a visual portrayal of your advancement. You probably won't see changes in the mirror consistently; however photographs required weeks or months separated can show a sensational contrast.

Journaling

Keeping a diary of your food consumption, sleep, state of mind, and different elements can assist you with seeing examples and make associations between your propensities and your advancement.

Applications and Technology

There are numerous applications and technology accessible that can follow your food consumption, steps, sleep, from there, the sky's the limit. These can give a nitty gritty image of your propensities and progress.

Recollect consistency is vital

It isn't not difficult to get thinner. It takes a ton of difficult work and all the more significantly, everything revolves around consistency. While following your weight reduction progress might give you a lift, considering that you have gained incredible outcomes, don't get unsettled in the event that you see no improvement.

Everyone is unique and keeping in mind that certain individuals might get results right away, others might need to work harder. At the end of the day, your commitment and assurance will prove to be fruitful, if you stay on track.

CHAPTER 9

CONCLUSION

In the journey of this book, we have analyzed different procedures that emphasize diet, way of life changes, and exceptional strategies to accomplish weight reduction and flat tummy. The objective was to give a practical and feasible structure that doesn't depend on demanding activity, but instead on careful decisions and propensities.

The methods outlined in this book are designed to be incorporated into your daily routine with ease. They are not quick fixes, but sustainable changes that can lead to long-term results. Remember, the key to success is consistency. It's about making small, manageable changes to your diet and lifestyle that you can stick to in the long run.

We've debunked the myth that exercise is the only way to lose weight and get a flat tummy. While exercise is beneficial for overall health and fitness, it's not the only factor. Your diet, sleep, stress levels and hydration also play crucial roles. By focusing on these aspects, you can achieve your weight loss goals and maintain a flat tummy without stepping foot in a gym.

Remember, every step, no matter how small, brings you closer to your goal. Be patient with yourself, celebrate your progress, and don't be discouraged by setbacks.

There will be twists and turns on your path, but with the knowledge and insights you've gained here, you'll be able to navigate with resilience and purpose. Your journey is unique. I hope your journey is filled with self-discovery, growth, and most importantly, a dedication to the long-term well-being that results from a positive connection with your health.

I'm wishing you good health, energy, and a bright future full of the benefits of living a well-rounded life.

www.ingramcontent.com/pod-product-compliance
Lightning Source LLC
Chambersburg PA
CBHW050828250726
48653CB00006B/2493